WORKOUT GUIDE

HOW TO USE HOUSEHOLD ITEMS AS EXERCISE EQUIPMENTS

A.D RAMS

Contents

CHAPTER ONE

INTRODUCTION

The idea of exercising at home has been very popular in recent years, and with good cause. For those with hectic schedules, restricted access to fitness centers, or a simple preference for ease, at-home exercise sessions are a useful way to maintain physical fitness. You might not always have access to standard exercise equipment, though. Thankfully, your home has a plethora of imaginative possibilities. You can turn your living room into an inexpensive gym without compromising on efficacy by upcycling common household objects.

We'll look at how to use common household objects as exercise equipment in this tutorial, providing a range of workouts and exercises suitable for varying fitness levels and objectives. You will learn how to get the most out of the equipment you already have at home, from basic bodyweight exercises to more difficult resistance training. Using everyday objects as training equipment opens up a world of options for reaching your fitness objectives from the comfort of your own home, regardless of your level of experience or desire for new challenges as an athlete.

Now let's get started and examine the adaptability, inventiveness, and efficiency of utilizing common household objects to improve your at-home exercises and reach new levels of fitness.

Exercise's Significance for Health and Well-Being

Exercise has a significant impact on many facets of physical, mental, and emotional fitness, and is essential for fostering general health and well-being. For your health and well-being, exercise is crucial for the following reasons:

Advantages for Physical Health:

Enhances Cardiovascular Health: Frequent exercise lowers blood pressure, increases blood circulation, and strengthens the heart muscle, all of which lower the risk of heart disease and stroke.

Enhances Muscle Growth, Strength, and Endurance: Exercise helps to build stronger, more flexible muscles that help with posture, balance, and mobility. This lowers the chance of accidents and falls.

Helps with Weight Management: Exercise is a great way to lose weight, maintain weight, and improve body composition because it increases metabolism, controls hunger, and burns calories.

Boosts Bone Density: By encouraging bone development and density, weight-bearing activities like jogging, walking, and resistance training lower the risk of osteoporosis and fractures.

Enhances Immune Function: Frequent exercise builds immunity, lowering the risk of infections and diseases and encouraging a quicker recovery from sickness.

Advantages for Mental Health:

Lessens tension and Anxiety: Exercise causes the production of endorphins, which are happy-making and calming neurotransmitters that lessen tension, anxiety, and sadness.

Boosts Mood and Self-esteem: By encouraging a sense of empowerment, mastery, and accomplishment, physical activity raises mood, self-esteem, and confidence levels.

Enhances Cognitive performance: By boosting neuroplasticity, increasing blood flow to the brain, and lowering the risk of dementia and cognitive decline, exercise improves memory, focus, and cognitive performance.

Enhances Sleep Quality: By controlling circadian cycles, lowering insomnia, and encouraging relaxation, regular exercise enhances both the quality and length of sleep.

Advantages for Emotional Well-being:

Enhances Coping Skills: Exercise promotes resilience, emotional balance, and a sense of control as a healthy coping strategy for handling stress, negative emotions, and life's obstacles.

Promotes Social Connections: Taking part in sports, outdoor activities, or group exercise courses promotes camaraderie, a sense of belonging, and social connections that lessen feelings of isolation and loneliness.

Encourages Mindfulness and Relaxation: Exercises that increase awareness, relaxation, and a sense of present-moment awareness, such as yoga, tai chi, or walking in the outdoors, can help clear the mind and foster inner calm.

Maintaining the best possible physical, mental, and emotional health and well-being requires regular exercise. There are many advantages to engaging in regular physical activity that lead to a life that is healthier, happier, and more satisfying. Unlocking the transforming power of exercise for your overall well-being requires finding methods to stay active, whether it's through regular movement, recreational activities, or scheduled training.

Accessing Conventional Exercise Equipment Presents Difficulties

For those who want to exercise regularly, getting access to typical exercise equipment like machines, free weights, or specialist gym gear can present a number of obstacles. The following are some typical obstacles to obtaining conventional exercise equipment:

Cost: Buying traditional exercise equipment, especially high-quality machines or weightlifting gear, may be costly. For many people, especially those on a tight budget, the initial outlay needed to set up a home gym or buy a gym membership with access to a large selection of equipment may be prohibitive.

Space Restrictions: Conventional workout equipment frequently needs a specific area to be used and stored. Not everyone has the benefit of a large home or access to a fitness center with enough room for large equipment setups or bulky machines. It can be difficult to fit heavy workout equipment or store free weights and supplies in a small space.

Accessibility: People who live in isolated or rural locations with few fitness centers nearby may have restricted access to traditional workout equipment. Moreover, access to exercise equipment that is not made to meet their needs may be hampered for those with physical disabilities or mobility issues.

Time Restraints: Having a regular workout program and accessing gym facilities during peak hours can be difficult due to busy schedules and time limits. Prolonged travels to the fitness center or waiting for equipment to become available may deter people from exercising on a regular basis.

Maintenance and Upkeep: To maintain safe and efficient operation, traditional workout equipment needs to undergo routine maintenance and upkeep. This could entail doing repairs on broken equipment, cleaning, lubricating moving parts, and replacing worn-out parts. Over time, improper maintenance of exercise equipment can jeopardize both its functionality and safety.

Fear and Ignorance: The intricacy of conventional exercise equipment can intimidate or overwhelm some people, particularly if they are not familiar with correct use or technique. People may be discouraged from adding equipment into their workout program if they lack the necessary information or assistance in using it properly.

Preference for Variety: To keep their workouts interesting and fun, some people may prefer a range of exercise modalities and activities, even while typical exercise equipment can offer good workouts. Their capacity to experiment with various types of physical activity may be limited if they don't have access to a wide variety of fitness classes or equipment.

Risk of damage: If people do not receive enough education or supervision on technique and safety considerations, improper use of traditional exercise equipment, especially free weights or resistance machines, can raise the risk of damage. At fitness centers, inadequate supervision or a staff devoid of expertise might exacerbate this risk.

All things considered, while traditional exercise equipment can provide a host of advantages for physical fitness and well-being, certain people may find access and use restricted by a variety of obstacles. Fortunately, there are substitutes that may be used to stay active and in shape. Some of these substitutes include bodyweight exercises, functional training, and repurposing household items as exercise equipment.

Safety Procedures and Directives

Prioritizing safety is crucial while utilizing everyday objects as training equipment in order to avoid accidents and guarantee productive workouts. The following are some safety measures and recommendations to abide by:

Examine Everything: Make sure all household things are strong, stable, and free of flaws or problems that could jeopardize safety before utilizing them for exercise. Look for indications of deterioration, missing components, or sharp edges that could cut someone while in use.

CHAPTER TWO

Choose the Right Items: Make sure the home objects you choose will support your body weight or resistance needs securely and are appropriate for the activities you intend to conduct. When exercising, stay away from using objects that are excessively heavy, unstable, or delicate.

Employ Correct Form and Technique: To reduce the chance of injury and increase efficacy, use correct form and technique for every exercise. Keep an eye on your alignment, posture, and movement mechanics. Steer clear of momentum-based or jerky motions that could put strain on your joints or muscles.

Start Slowly and Increase Gradually: If you're new to exercising with household goods, especially if you're not comfortable with the movements, start with lower resistance or lower intensity exercises. As your strength and confidence grow, gradually increase the resistance, repetitions, or complexity of the exercises.

Warm Up Correctly: Give careful consideration to a warm-up regimen before to beginning an exercise session in order to prime your muscles, joints, and cardiovascular system for action. For increased flexibility and blood flow, incorporate dynamic stretches, mobility exercises, and light cardio.

Employ Padding or Cushioning: To protect your skin and joints, use padding or cushioning while utilizing household goods that could put pressure or discomfort on your body, such as hard surfaces or edges. If necessary, place a yoga mat, towel, or exercise mat between the object and your skin, or beneath your body.

Drink lots of water before, during, and after your workout to stay hydrated and avoid dehydration. Also, remember to take breaks. Between workouts or sets, take regular pauses to recover, regain your breath, and avoid overdoing it.

Listen to Your Body: During exercise, pay attention to how your body feels and modify your technique or intensity accordingly. If an activity is causing you pain, discomfort, or dizziness, stop doing it and get help from a doctor if needed.

Clear Surrounding Area: To avoid mishaps or collisions with surrounding objects or furniture, make sure there is enough room and clearance around you when utilizing household goods for exercise. Eliminate any risks or obstructions that could cause someone to trip and fall.

Seek Professional Advice: Consult a certified fitness expert or personal trainer for advice if you're unclear about the safest and most efficient ways to employ common home objects for workout. They may offer you advice, direction, and customized recommendations to help you safely reach your fitness objectives.

You can utilize common household items as exercise equipment to enjoy safe, injury-free exercises as long as you take the necessary safety precautions and recommendations. Prioritize safety above all else, pay attention to your body, and see a doctor before beginning a new fitness regimen if you have any underlying medical illnesses or concerns.

Exercises for the Heart

Cardiovascular workouts are crucial for enhancing general fitness, burning calories, and heart health. Even if you don't have easy access to standard cardio equipment like ellipticals, stationary bikes, or treadmills at home, you can still work out your heart with everyday objects.

Using common household items as exercise equipment, try these cardiovascular exercises:

Jump Rope: Needing little room and equipment, jumping rope is an incredibly efficient cardio workout. You can either improvise with a piece of rope or cable or use a conventional jump rope. Agility, cardiovascular endurance, and coordination can all be enhanced by jumping rope.

Exercises involving stair climbing: Make use of the staircase in your house. Just keep going up and down the steps while walking, running, or jogging to increase your heart rate and strengthen your lower body muscles. Stair sprints or climbing steps two at a time are good ways to up the intensity.

Step-Ups: To execute step-ups, utilize a strong household item such as a low stool, step stool, or the lowest step of a staircase. Place one foot on the platform, step up to meet it with the other, and then step back down. To equally train both sides, switch up the leading legs.

High Knees: While running or marching in place, stay still and raise your knees as high as you can. To boost intensity, pump your arms in sync with your legs. High knees can be done as a circuit exercise or for a predetermined amount of time.

Burpees: A full-body exercise that blends strength and cardio training is the burpee. Commence in a standing posture, descend into a squat, plant your hands on the ground, leap backwards into a plank position, execute a push-up, leap backwards into your hands, and leap skywards with force. For a workout that is high in cardio, repeat continually.

Mountain Climbers: Start in the plank position, with your body in a straight line from your head to your heels and your hands directly beneath your shoulders. Maintaining an engaged core, alternate between bringing your knees to your chest in a running motion. Make rapid movements to increase your heart rate.

Squat Jumps: To increase your heart rate and tone your lower body muscles, perform squat jumps. Begin in a squat, then leap skyward with great force, raising your arms above your head.

Gently return to the squat position and repeat for the designated number of repetitions or duration.

Dancing: For a fun and efficient cardio workout, turn on your favorite music and dance about your living room. Include a variety of dance steps to keep your body moving and your heart rate elevated, such as shuffles, twists, kicks, and jumping jacks.

Shadow Boxing: Take a wide stance and alternate between jabs, crosses, hooks, and uppercuts when you toss punches into the air. To intensify, mimic boxing moves with your feet and torso while maintaining a constant beat.

Running or Jogging in Place: To raise your heart rate and burn calories when you have limited room, just run or jog in place. To simulate jogging outside, raise your legs high and swing your arms.

These cardiovascular workouts can effectively increase cardiovascular fitness, burn calories, and enhance general health since they employ common household items as exercise equipment. Combine these workouts to build a difficult and unique cardio program that suits your fitness level and objectives. To avoid injury and get the most out of your workout, always start out slowly, build up your intensity gradually, and pay attention to your body.

Exercises for Strength Training

Gaining muscle, gaining strength, and enhancing general functional fitness all depend on strength training. Even though you might not have access to standard gym equipment like dumbbells, barbells, and machines at home, you can still execute efficient strength training exercises with common household items acting as temporary equipment. Here are some strength training activities that you may perform using everyday household objects:

Bodyweight Squats: Squats work the quadriceps, hamstrings, and glutes, and are a great complex exercise for the lower body. Place your feet shoulder-width apart and squat, maintaining your knees in line with your toes and your chest raised, as though you were reclining in a chair.

Hold onto heavy household objects, such as gallon jugs filled with water or laundry detergent, to increase resistance.

Lunges: Lunges enhance stability and balance while working the quadriceps, hamstrings, glutes, and calves. Step one foot forward while keeping your feet together and bending both knees to drop yourself into a lunge. Repeat on the other side after pushing yourself back up to the starting position. To strengthen your resistance, hang onto common home objects like rice bags or canned goods.

Push-ups: A traditional upper body workout, push-ups work the triceps, shoulders, and chest. With your hands shoulder-width apart, begin in the plank position. Lower your body toward the floor while maintaining your elbows close to your sides. Return to the starting position by pushing, then repeat for the designated number of reps or duration. Push-ups can be made simpler by doing them on an incline with a strong household object, such as a bench or countertop.

Chair Dips: This exercise works the chest and core muscles as well as the triceps and shoulders. Hands on the front edge of a strong chair or bench, fingers pointing forward, while you sit on its edge. Step your feet out, bend your elbows to bring your body down to the floor, and then push yourself back up to the starting position.

Variations on the Plank: Planks are a great way to develop your shoulders, core, and stabilizing muscles. Laying down on your forearms and toes, perform conventional planks, maintaining a straight body from head to heels. Try plank jacks, side planks, or forearm planks with alternate shoulder taps to provide some variation.

Single-Leg Deadlifts: These exercises strengthen the lower back, glutes, and hamstrings while also enhancing stability and balance. Grasp a robust domestic object in one hand, such as a rucksack loaded with books or a gallon jug. Maintaining a straight back, descend the object towards the floor by bending your knee slightly and pivoting forward at the hips. Go back to the beginning and repeat with the other leg.

Rows: The latissimus dorsi and rhomboids are two muscles in the upper back that can be effectively targeted by rows. As resistance, utilize a robust household object, such as a packed bag or backpack. Lean forward at the hips, bending your knees slightly, and hold the object with both hands while extending your arms toward the ground. Squeeze your shoulder blades together as you pull the object towards your torso, then carefully lower it back down.

Calf Raises: These exercises, which focus on the calf muscles, can be done on a step, a staircase, or a sturdy household object to elevate yourself up. As you allow your heels to drop toward the floor, stand with the balls of your feet resting on the edge of the step or object. Elevate your heels as high as you can by pressing through the balls of your feet, then carefully descend back down.

CHAPTER THREE

Wall Sits: This isometric exercise works the glutes, hamstrings, and quads. Place your back against a strong wall and sit down, keeping your knees bent at a 90-degree angle and your thighs parallel to the floor. Keep your legs in this position for a predetermined amount of time, making sure to use them.

Backpack Squats: To add resistance to squats, lunges, or other lower body workouts, stuff a backpack with heavy books, canned goods, or water bottles. To make the workouts harder and help you gain strength, wear the backpack firmly on your back.

These strength training routines that employ common home objects as exercise equipment can offer efficient workouts to boost strength, develop muscle, and enhance general fitness. If you're new to strength training, start with lower resistance or bodyweight exercises and work your way up to more intensity and resistance as you gain strength and proficiency. Before beginning a new fitness program, always remember to maintain appropriate form, pay attention to your body, and see a healthcare provider if you have any underlying health disorders or concerns.

Exercises for Flexibility and Mobility

Enhancing overall movement quality, avoiding accidents, and preserving joint health all depend on increased flexibility and mobility. Even while you might not have access to standard stretching tools like foam rollers or yoga blocks at home, you can still do efficient flexibility and mobility exercises with everyday household items. The following workouts can be performed with household items acting as temporary equipment:

Towel Stretch: To target different muscle areas, practice a range of stretches using a bath towel or belt. To stretch the hamstring, for instance, lie on your back, wrap the towel over one foot, and then slowly draw the leg toward your chest. Stretching your quadriceps and shoulders while standing or lying down is another way you can utilize the towel.

Chair Yoga: As you execute yoga poses that increase flexibility and mobility, use a firm chair to support your balance and stability. To stretch the hamstrings, hips, and spine, perform supported lunges, seated twists, and forward folds using the chair. Chair yoga may be adjusted to match mobility constraints and is appropriate for people of all fitness levels.

Stretching on a Staircase: Use a staircase in your house to work your hamstrings, hip flexors, and calves. To lengthen your calves, stand on the bottom step with the balls of your feet resting on the edge. Then, let your heels fall toward the floor. To extend the stretch, slowly lean forward while holding onto the railing for support.

Support with Pillow or Cushion: When performing floor stretches and yoga poses, support your body using pillows or cushions. For support and cushioning during hip openers, spinal twists, or supine stretches, place cushions beneath your knees or hips. You may adjust the stiffness and height of the pillows to make the stretch as comfortable as possible.

Door Frame Stretch: To stretch your upper back, shoulders, and chest, use a door frame. Place your elbows on the door frame and stand facing the door frame with your arms bent at a 90-degree angle. To feel a stretch over your shoulders and chest, gently lean forward. Alternatively, you can lean forward and place one hand on each side of the door frame to conduct a doorway chest stretch.

Water Bottles or Cans for Weighted Stretches: To deepen stretches and increase flexibility, use water bottles, canned goods, or other common home items as temporary weights. To increase resistance and stretch intensity, hold onto the items while you conduct seated or standing stretches. To intensify the stretch in the front of the thigh, for instance, hold a water bottle in each hand while stretching your quadriceps while standing.

Blanket or Towel for Joint Mobility: When performing kneeling or sitting mobility exercises, place a folded blanket or towel between your knees to cushion them or to support you. When performing sitting spinal twists or kneeling hip circles, place the blanket under your knees to ease discomfort and promote more fluid movement.

Wall Support for Standing Stretches: When doing standing stretches that work the quadriceps, hamstrings, and calves, use a wall for stability and support. Place your hands shoulder-height on the wall as you face the wall, then take a step back with your foot to form a lunge. Feel the calf and hamstring muscles in your back leg stretch as you gently lean forward.

Book or Block for Prop Support: During yoga or stretching activities, use books, blocks, or other sturdy objects as props to support your body. To offer support and ensure correct alignment, place the prop beneath your hands or forehead during forward folds, or under your hips during sitting stretches.

Make Your Own Foam Roller: For self-myofascial release, tightly roll up a towel or blanket to make a makeshift foam roller. Place the rolled-up towel under tense or aching muscles, including the calves, hips, or upper back. To provide pressure and alleviate tension in the muscles and fascia, slowly roll back and forth.

By utilizing common home items as workout equipment, these flexibility and mobility exercises can help increase joint range of motion, lessen muscle stiffness, and improve the overall quality of movement. Include these exercises in your daily regimen to improve joint health, flexibility, and mobility. Never forget to stretch slowly and softly, avoiding any motions that hurt or are uncomfortable. Before beginning a new stretching or mobility program, see a healthcare professional if you have any current injuries or illnesses.

Exercises for Balance and Function

For the purpose of enhancing stability, coordination, and movement efficiency in daily tasks, functional training and balancing exercises are crucial. Even though you might not have access to standard gym equipment like stability balls or balance boards at home, you can still do efficient functional training and balancing exercises with everyday household items. The following workouts can be performed with household items acting as temporary equipment:

Single-Leg Balance: For a predetermined amount of time, stand on one leg and raise the other leg off the ground to maintain balance. If support is required, utilize a strong household object like a chair or countertop. Throughout the workout, pay attention to maintaining your body's stability and your core. Repeat after switching legs.

Heel-to-Toe Walking: Step forward in a straight line, placing one foot in front of the other, contacting heel to toe. Practice heel-to-toe walking on a designated track in your house, like a hallway or open area, to help with balance and coordination.

Cushion or Pillow Balance: To test your stability and balance, stand on a cushion or pillow that is placed on the ground. For extra challenge, begin standing on one foot after placing both feet on the cushion. If you need assistance, use a nearby wall or piece of substantial furniture.

Plank variants: Engage in plank variants that test your core strength and stability. To strengthen stabilizing muscles and enhance balance, try plank rotations, side planks, and forearm planks with leg lifts. To provide comfort and padding, use a towel or yoga mat.

Toe Taps: Take a stand with your back to a low-hanging object in your home, like a book stack. Step up one foot, lightly tap your toes on the step or object, and then step back down to the beginning position. For repetitions, switch up your feet, paying attention to your balance and control the entire time.

Chair Squats: For squatting workouts, utilize a solid chair or a low object from around the house as your target. Place your feet hip-width apart in front of the chair, stoop down so that you appear to be sitting back into it, and then stand back up. When necessary, use the chair to provide stability and support; eventually, lessen your reliance on it.

Book Stack Lunge: Raise a heavy object from around the house or a stack of books in front of your chest using both hands. Maintaining the stability of the book stack, take a single stride back into a lunge position. Bending both knees, lower your body toward the ground and then rise back to the starting position. Continue on the opposite side.

Resistance Training with a Towel or Belt: For upper body and core movements, use a towel or belt. Exercises like rows, bicep curls, and tricep extensions can be done while holding one end of the towel in each hand. To keep your balance and support your body during the exercises, contract your core muscles.

Broomstick balancing: Use both hands to hold a broom or mop handle horizontally in front of your body. Keep the broomstick level and steady by balancing it on your palms and holding it there for a predetermined amount of time. Close your eyes and move forward by standing on one leg and keeping the broomstick balanced.

Step-Up Variations: For step-up exercises, utilize a strong household object such as the bottom step of a staircase or a low stool. Place one foot on the object and then raise the other to meet it. Retrace your steps and repeat for as long as necessary. If support is required, use a wall or railing that is close by.

To enhance your stability, coordination, and movement control, incorporate these functional training and balance exercises with everyday household items into your regular exercise regimen. As you gain strength and confidence, gradually raise the difficulty of the exercises to match your current level of fitness. When performing any workout, pay close attention to form, control, and awareness to increase efficiency and lower chance of injury. Before beginning a new fitness regimen, get advice from a healthcare professional if you have any current illnesses or injuries.

Establishing a Workout Program at Home

You don't need a gym membership or specialist equipment to keep active and fit by using common household items into a home workout regimen. Here's how to use everyday home objects to build a thorough at-home fitness routine:

Evaluate Your Fitness Objectives: Establish your objectives for fitness, be they increasing flexibility, strengthening muscles, strengthening cardiovascular systems, or boosting general fitness. Your home workout routine's structure and content will be determined by your goals.

Create a Well-Balanced Exercise Program: Include a range of exercises that focus on various muscle groups and aspects of fitness, such as cardio, strength, flexibility, and balance. Strive for a well-rounded fitness regimen that include both aerobic and resistance training.

Choosing Home Goods for Resistance Training: Opt for everyday objects that can be repurposed as temporary training apparatuses for resistance training. Water bottles, canned goods, book-filled backpacks, chairs, stairs, and walls for stability are a few examples.

Warm-Up: To get your muscles, joints, and cardiovascular system ready for exercise, begin your workout with a vigorous warm-up. Spend five to ten minutes on exercises including dynamic stretches, arm circles, leg swings, and stationary running.

Strength Training Exercises: Use common home items as resistance in a range of strength training exercises that focus on main muscle groups. Use water bottles, canned foods, or bags as weights for workouts including squats, lunges, push-ups, rows, overhead presses, and planks. For every exercise, try to do two to three sets of eight to twelve reps.

Incorporate cardiovascular exercises into your routine to increase heart rate and enhance cardiovascular health. Spend twenty to thirty minutes doing exercises like jumping jacks, high knees, burpees, mountain climbers, stair climbing, or dancing to your favorite music. To maintain a lively and interesting workout, switch up the exercises.

workouts for Flexibility and Mobility: Combine workouts for flexibility and mobility to enhance joint range of motion, ease tense muscles, and ward against injuries. Use chairs, walls, and towels as well as other household items to provide support when performing stretches that target main muscle groups. Stretch for 15 to 30 seconds, then repeat two or three times.

Exercises for Balance and Stability: Include exercises for balance and stability to improve core strength, proprioception, and coordination. To test your stability and control, try single-leg balancing, heel-to-toe walks, cushion or pillow balances, and chair squats.

Stretch and cool down: Finish your workout with a cooldown to let your heart rate gradually drop and aid in recuperation. To increase flexibility and reduce discomfort in your muscles, perform static stretches that focus on your main muscle groups. For 15 to 30 seconds, hold each stretch while concentrating on relaxing and deep breathing.

Track Your Progress: Keep a log of the length, intensity, and perceived exertion of your workouts to monitor your progress over time. Depending on your fitness objectives, preferences, and progress, modify your at-home exercise program as necessary.

Remain Consistent: To keep up your fitness and make progress, try to work out three to five times a week. To promote consistency, plan your workouts for convenient times and set aside a specific area in your house for it.

By following these guidelines, you can use common household items as exercise equipment to create a successful at-home workout routine. In order to optimize outcomes and reduce the chance of injury, always remember to put safety, good form, and gradual progression first. Seek advice and support from a fitness expert or personal trainer if you're unclear of how to carry out specific exercises or develop a customized training schedule.

Summary

In summary, everyday objects can be used as adaptable and powerful exercise equipment, enabling you to design demanding workouts and maintain your fitness level without the need for specialized equipment or a gym membership. Household items offer endless possibilities for imaginative and dynamic workouts, whether your goals are to increase strength, cardiovascular health, flexibility, or balance and stability. Commonplace objects such as chairs, walls, water bottles, towels, and stairs can be repurposed to target all major muscle groups, raise heart rate, improve flexibility, and improve overall fitness.

The secret to using everyday objects as workout equipment is to be inventive, resourceful, and persistent. You can design a well-rounded exercise program that meets your fitness objectives and keeps you inspired and involved by mixing up the exercises and movements in your routine. Keep in mind that the best ways to reduce the chance of injury and increase outcomes are to prioritize safety, good form, and gradual progression.

Whether you're a beginner looking to kickstart your fitness journey or a seasoned athlete seeking new challenges, harnessing the power of household items as exercise equipment opens up a world of possibilities for achieving your health and fitness goals from the comfort of your own home. So use common household items as your reliable exercise partners and get creative, have fun, and enjoy the journey to a healthier, stronger, and more resilient you.

THE END